20 Minutes Keto Diet Book

Fast and Easy Keto Recipes For Every Day with a 14-Day Starter Meal Plan

Mike H. Ward

TABLE OF CONTENTS

Mains 41

VEGETARIAN 42

MEAT 60

EXCLUSIVE BONUS

40 Weight Loss Recipes

&

14 Days Meal Plan

Scan the QR-Code and receive
the FREE download:

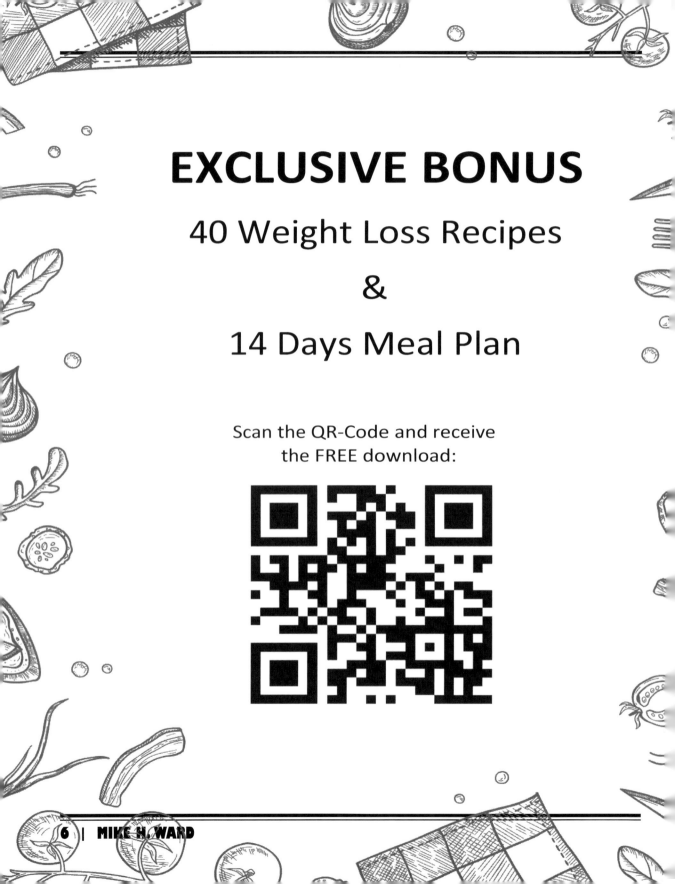

Welcome to 'The 20 Minutes Keto Diet Book'

In the coming pages you'll find 30+ new and exciting keto recipes that will leave you drooling for more, and all of them are prepared in 20 minutes or less!

Find out more about what the Keto diet involves, and kickstart your keto journey using our BONUS 14-day keto starter meal plan

Transform into the best version of yourself by going keto...today!

WHAT IS THE KETO DIET?

The keto, or ketogenic, diet is a low-carb, high-fat diet that is designed to induce a natural metabolic change. This change is to put the body into ketosis; a metabolic state whereby fat is burned for energy instead of glucose, aka carbohydrates. The body will naturally enter a stage of ketosis after 3-5 days, if consuming less than 50g of carbohydrates per day.

In order to maintain optimal body and mental functioning it is necessary to balance the lowered carbohydrate intake with an increased fat intake- hence the diet being high-fat. When adopting the keto diet, it is recommended to have 70%-80% of your overall calorific intake coming from fat sources.

Unlike many 'traditional' diets, calorie counting is advised **against** on the keto diet. The nature of the keto diet is to focus on micro and macro nutrients rather than calories, and the high-fat nature of the diet greatly increases calorie numbers. Fat contains roughly 9 kcal/gram, whereas carbohydrates and proteins contain only 4 kcal/gram. Therefore, by substituting fats for carbohydrates daily calories are inevitably much higher.

Over 30 recent scientific studies have discovered that, especially in comparison to other diets, the keto diet assists effective, sustainable, and medically sound weight loss.

How does ketosis work?

Ketosis works by inducing a deviation from the natural metabolic state, a process achieved by limiting carbohydrate intake. The body is forced to find an alternative energy source, and so responds to this need for energy by producing ketones, an acidic chemical body designed to break down fat molecules as an alternative energy source. Ketones will break down dietary fat and body fat, in order to provide a steady supply of fuel to the body.

Because a healthy alternative energy is supplied (fat) the keto diet can be followed for an indefinite period of time. Unlike some diets the keto plan avoids fasting or restriction, and facilitates a steady trajectory of weight loss, instead of the classic 'yo-yo dieting' trap.

WHAT ARE THE BENEFITS OF THE KETO DIET?

There are numerous proven health benefits of the keto diet aside from the weight loss it is famed for.

Those suffering with specific medical conditions such as epilepsy, Alzheimer's, Parkinson's disease, and Type 2 diabetes are recommended to adopt the keto diet due to its positive impact upon such conditions. Management or minimisation of symptoms is a huge benefit that the keto diet facilitates.

On a day to day basis the keto diet is useful for the following:

- Sustainable weight loss
- Increased energy
- Increased mental functioning- focus, concentration, and overall clarity
- Maintaining muscle mass
- Heightened physical performance
- Improved skin condition, in particular the effects of acne
- Settling of persistent stomach issues, such as IBS, gas, and cramping
- Appetite regulator and feelings of increased satiety
- Reduced cravings for high carbohydrate foods
- A lowered risk of heart disease
  - -Improved cholesterol profile
  - -Improved blood sugar levels
  - -Improved insulin levels
  - -Improved blood pressure

WILL MY HEALTH IMPROVE ON THE KETO DIET ALONE?

As with any diet, to really reap the benefits simply changing up your food won't work miracles- for optimum results a whole lifestyle shift is recommended. The best way to lose weight and adopt a healthier lifestyle is to first assess where you struggle:

- Do you snack excessively?
- Do you comfort eat?
- Do you restrict your food and then end up bingeing?
- Do you exercise regularly?
- Do you lead a life conducive to overall wellness?

By first asking yourself these questions you can figure out what you're seeking by adopting the keto diet. When used alongside moderate exercise and mindfulness the keto diet can seem to work wonders... but that isn't the case. It is valuing yourself enough to want the best for yourself that is the real miracle.

What foods can and can't be eaten?

Cutting out carbohydrates sounds a lot harder than it is- there's a great smorgasbord of low-carb culinary delights out there!

As a general guide it is best to avoid:

- Any foods that are artificially sweetened or flavoured
- Foods that are highly processed and containing 'hidden' ingredients
- Low fat products
- Grains
- Starchy vegetables (the 'tuber' food group)
- Fruits (excluding berries in small quantities)
- Legumes

Thankfully, there are loads of alternatives now available for any dietary requirements. Low carbohydrate alternatives for sugars, flours, and other traditionally high carbohydrate foods are readily available at specialist food stores and supermarkets, and some can even be made at home. Even those with a sweet tooth will still be able to treat themselves in a keto approved way!

A typical keto diet is full of healthy fats, meats, poultry, dairy products, certain fruits, and plenty of vegetables, but as your personal keto journey unfurls you'll discover the best way to make it work for you.

What are 'Macros'?

Macros, or macronutrients, is another term associated with the keto diet. Macros refer to where your calories are coming from, and therefore how to calculate the ideal keto plan for yourself.

The ideal macro ratio to initiate ketosis is understood to be:

> **70%** of calories from *fat*   (9kcal/g)
>
> **25%** of calories from *protein*   (4kcal/g)
>
> **5%** of calories from *carbohydrates*   (4kcal/g)

These figures can vary greatly from individual to individual, so you must first figure out your personal daily macro requirements. Do this by working out your daily calorific needs using an online tool or with a caloric calculator app.

Caloric needs vary greatly dependent upon factors such as age, gender, current eight, goal weight, activity levels, etc., so it is best to take some time to work out what you individually need for optimum results.

WHAT ARE 'NET CARBS'?

You will hear the term 'net carbs' time and time again on your keto journey. This term refers to the carbohydrates that the body is capable of digesting- the ones that don't present themselves as fibrous roughage. This dietary fibre is essential to ensure a healthy gut and bowel, but it isn't digested or absorbed by your body, and therefore these carbohydrates do not count as part of your overall daily carbohydrate intake.

It's easy to calculate your net carbs when you understand this point. Take, for example, a large tomato- roughly 60g.

> The **total carbohydrates** within this tomato is 2.4g
>
> The **dietary fibre** within this tomato is 0.7g
>
> Therefore, the **net carbs** will be 2.4g − 0.7g = 1.7g

If you're ever unsure of nutritional information first distinguish between the overall carbohydrates and the net carbohydrates- remember this formula in order to prevent restricting yourself further, or shying away from foods that appear too high in carbohydrates- the likelihood is that when dietary fibre is take into account the carbohydrate count will significantly decrease.

How do I know how many carbohydrates I can eat?

There are roughly 3 levels of carbohydrate restrictions based on net carbs per day. These levels are in line with the definition that **a low carb diet is a consumption of less than 130g of carbohydrates per day, or 20% of energy from carbohydrates**. These levels can be understood as:

Ketogenic	<20 g/day	4% energy
Moderate low carb	20-50 g/day	4-10% energy
Max low carb	50-130 g/day	10-20% energy

Carbohydrate intake varies from person to person, but the idea is to start by not exceeding 50g of carbohydrates a day, and as your body adapts slowly adjusting and lowering that number until you are consuming less than 20g of carbohydrates in a day.

As time goes by and you grow more confident in your self and your body, we hope that counting every micro, macro, carb or calorie will no longer be necessary. By finding recipes that you trust and enjoy, and slowly building up your knowledge of what is keto, what isn't keto, what can be made to suit keto etc. you'll be able to maintain your new ketogenic lifestyle independently.

CAN I EVER HAVE A 'CHEAT' DAY?

A cheat day is a day within a diet regime that the individual is permitted to disregard their diet guidelines and eat what they like. Some people adopt this mentality with the keto diet, others don't- it's up to you. There are pros to cheat days and there are cons, as is with everything in life. The recipes you will find within this book and other keto recipes tend to be variations of other foods, allowing you to still eat classic bread, sweets, and sugar, but in a keto friendly way. For some people however, these adapted alternatives don't hit the spot, and that's where cheat days come in.

Motivations for cheating are a big tell as to whether your cheating is legitimate or not- are you being 'polite'? Are you acting impulsively? Did you accidentally go over your daily carbohydrate allowance and are now throwing caution to the wind? Improper motivation to justify a cheat day indicates whether you are committed or not to the keto lifestyle.

On the other hand, if your motivation is to be realistic and know you can't be perfect on your keto diet, if there's a special occasion and you want to join in, or other reasons that factor in a deliberate intention and plan to 'cheat' then it may work out well for you. Never having a slice of cake again may put you off pursuing a keto lifestyle, and so by factoring in such treats in moderation you are actually planning for the long term, and avoiding a mindset of rigid deprivation.

There are warnings that come with cheating. Your body may once again crave high carb foods or react badly to a sudden sugar spike. You may experience sudden weight gain and reduced motivation. Feelings of guilt and shame may lead you back to a sugar addiction you fought so hard to overcome...

There's a whole host of unwanted results that come alongside cheat days, but there are also benefits, and the choice is up to you. Consult with your keto comrades to learn of their experiences and advice in order to make an informed decision that has your best interest at heart.

ARE THERE ANY SIDE EFFECTS I NEED TO BE AWARE OF?

Many people experience an initial weight loss of 1-2kg within the first week, but this tends to be losing weight from water stored within the body. As your body and metabolism adapts your weight loss trajectory will change; on average 0.5kg per week, but once your optimum body weight is reached results are likely to slow drastically or change to weight maintenance.

Remember that continuous weight loss is not sustainable. The keto diet is a tool to achieve a healthy body and lifestyle. Once this has materialised the diet can either be followed for maintenance, or can be adapted to allow a higher daily carbohydrate limit. This is up to personal preference.

When adopting the keto diet it is also common to experience the 'keto flu'. This is the result of your body adjusting and entering ketosis. This is perfectly normal, but if your symptoms continue for an extended period of time it is advised to seek medical help. Some of the symptoms of the keto flu include:

- Disrupted sleep
- Fatigue
- Reduced concentration
- Irritability
- Changes in bowel movements- constipation or diarrhoea
- Bad breath

Because of the potential to fall victim to these side effects a gradual transition is recommended. This will not only lessen symptoms, but also allow you to grow your confidence and knowledge at a pace that works for you.

The keto diet is a manipulation of normal bodily functioning, and therefore should always be undertaken with caution. Be sure to research thoroughly and consult with others prior to committing to this shift.

There is also a low risk of entering 'ketoacidosis' if the diet is not properly undertaken and monitored. Ketoacidosis is a build up of ketones, and a dangerous increase in the acidity of the blood- this is often the effect of diabetes, alcoholism, overactive thyroid disorders, excessive exercise, and starvation. Symptoms of ketoacidosis resemble those of the keto flu, but more severe, and with additional symptoms such as trouble breathing, stomach pains, and throwing up. If you feel you are experiencing these symptoms seek medical advice immediately.

Breakfast

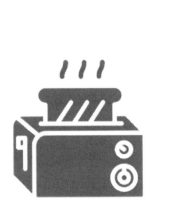

Egg and Bacon Avocado Boats

SERVES	4
CARBOHYDRATES	12G
PROTEIN	20G
FAT	36G
CALORIES	440

INGREDIENTS

- 4 ripe avocados
- 8 medium eggs
- 6 bacon rashers
- Chilli flakes to taste
- Salt and pepper to season

DIRECTIONS

1. Preheat your oven to 180C // 350F. Prepare your avocados by halving and stoning each, and then scooping out some flesh from each half so that the remaining flesh is left as a 1cm border

2. Place your prepared avocados into a large baking dish and crack an egg into each of the hollows. Season with salt and pepper, and sprinkle over your chilli flakes, before placing into the preheated oven

3. As your avocados cook dice your bacon rashers and place them into a large oiled frying pan over a high heat. Fry your bacon until crisp and browned before transferring onto a paper towel lined plate

4. After 15-20 minutes your avocados should be cooked- the whites should be firm, and the yolks should still be runny. Remove them from the oven and transfer to plates. Sprinkle over your crispy bacon and serve

Eggs Benedict

SERVES	4
CARBOHYDRATES	3G
PROTEIN	16G
FAT	48G
CALORIES	522

INGREDIENTS

- 2 avocados
- 4 medium eggs
- 4 slices of smoked salmon
- 1 tsp white vinegar
- Freshly cracked black pepper

HOLLANDAISE

- 8 tbsp butter
- 3 egg yolks
- 3 tsp lemon juice
- Salt and pepper to taste

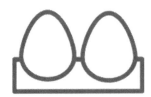

DIRECTIONS

1. Start by preparing your avocados- halve and destone the avocados, then remove the outer skin. Do this by cutting a slit at the top or bottom, and gently peeling away the skin with your fingers or a serving spoon

2. Begin making your hollandaise sauce by placing your butter in a microwave proof bowl and heating on high at 10 second intervals until the butter is melted, but not overheated and bubbling

3. Remove the bowl from the microwave and pour your melted butter, egg yolks, and lemon juice into a food processor. Blend on high until a thick, creamy sauce has formed. If you don't have a food processor then a hand-held blender will work equally well. Season your sauce with salt and pepper to taste

4. Whilst your sauce cools and settles poach your eggs. Bring a small pan of water to the boil, then reduce the heat to a steady simmer. Stir in your vinegar, then continue stirring to create a small whirlpool. Crack your eggs into separate saucers, then pour them one at a time into the pan

5. Cook each egg for 2-4 minutes, or until the white is set and the yolk is to your preference. Remove from the pan with a slotted spoon and place each egg onto your prepared avocado halves

6. Divide your hollandaise sauce between the 4 plates. Add a slice of smoked salmon to each plate, before topping with freshly cracked black pepper and serving

Huevos Rancheros

SERVES	4
CARBOHYDRATES	12G
PROTEIN	17G
FAT	46G
CALORIES	542

INGREDIENTS

- ◆ 125 ml // ½ c olive oil
- ◆ 1 yellow onion, diced
- ◆ 1 tbsp minced garlic
- ◆ 2 fresh jalapeno peppers, finely diced
- ◆ 500 ml // 2c tinned tomatoes
- ◆ 8 medium eggs
- ◆ 4 tbsp fresh coriander, chopped
- ◆ 1 large avocado, sliced
- ◆ Sprinkling of grated parmesan
- ◆ Salt and pepper to taste

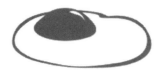

DIRECTIONS

1. Pour 3 tbsp of your oil into a saucepan over a medium heat. Sautee the onion, garlic, and jalapeno peppers for 5-10 minutes, or until they are all softened, and the onions are becoming translucent. Pour in your tinned tomatoes and reduce the heat for a steady simmer. Cover and leave to simmer until the mixture has formed a thick sauce

2. Whilst the sauce thickens heat your remaining oil on high in a large frying pan. Fry your eggs one at a time, cooking them until the white is set and the edges are crispy, but the yolk remains runny. Sprinkle over salt and pepper as they cook, then transfer to a paper towel lined plate once done

3. Divide the sauce between 4 serving dishes, and top each serving with 2 eggs. Sprinkle over your chopped coriander and grated parmesan, and add some sliced avocado to each dish. Top with freshly ground salt and pepper before serving

CAULIFLOWER TOAST

SERVES	6
CARBOHYDRATES	5G
PROTEIN	5G
FAT	4G
CALORIES	80

INGREDIENTS

- 1 medium/large cauliflower head
- 1 large egg
- 40 g // ½ c grated mozzarella
- ½ tbsp garlic powder
- Salt and pepper to taste

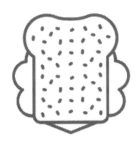

DIRECTIONS

1. Before starting preheat your oven to 200C // 400 F and grease or line a large baking tray

2. Break your cauliflower into florets and place these into a food processor. Pulse on high until your cauliflower is fully broken down and has a grainy, sand-like texture. Transfer the cauliflower into a large microwave proof bowl and heat on high for 7 minutes. Once heated pour your mixture into a tea towel or cheesecloth and squeeze firmly to remove any excess moisture

3. Pour your cauliflower back into your bowl and add in the egg, mozzarella, garlic powder, and salt and pepper to season. Use your hands or a wooden spoon to thoroughly combine everything

4. Divide your mixture into 6. Place each portion onto your prepared baking tray and shape to resemble a slice of toast. Transfer the tray into your preheated oven and bake for 12-15 minutes, or until the 'toast' is golden and crispy

5. Remove from the oven and serve immediately, topping with eggs, bacon, avocado, cheese, or whatever else may take your fancy

Everything Bagels

SERVES	8
CARBOHYDRATES	3.2G
PROTEIN	7.3G
FAT	12.7G
CALORIES	153

INGREDIENTS

- ◆ 240g // 3c grated mozzarella
- ◆ 5 tbsp cream cheese
- ◆ 2 large eggs (+ 1 lightly beaten for an egg wash)
- ◆ 200 g // 2c almond flour
- ◆ 3 tsp baking powder
- ◆ 4 tbsp 'everything bagel' seed mix or seasoning

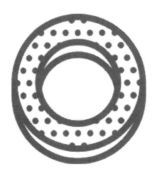

DIRECTIONS

1. Before starting preheat your oven to 200C // 400F, and line 2 medium baking trays with parchment paper

2. Place your grated mozzarella and cream cheese into a large, microwave safe bowl, and stir to roughly combine. Place into the microwave and heat on high for 30 second intervals, stirring in between. Continue until everything is melted and combined- roughly 2 minutes. Whilst the mixture heats, pour your almond flour and baking powder into a large bowl and whisk to combine

3. Spoon your cheese mixture into your flour and add your 2 eggs. Mix with a wooden spoon or your hands until everything is thoroughly combined, then divide this mixture into 8 portions. Roll each portion into a ball, then push your thumb through the centre of each to create a bagel shape

4. Transfer your bagels onto the prepared baking trays, then brush each with your egg wash and top with 'everything bagel' mix. Place into the preheated oven and bake for 20-25 minutes, or until golden brown with a firm exterior and cooked through

5. Allow your bagels to cool slightly before topping with your favourite fillings and serving

WAFFLES

SERVES	4
CARBOHYDRATES	15G
PROTEIN	11G
FAT	32G
CALORIES	307

INGREDIENTS

- ◆ 200g // 2c almond flour
- ◆ 50g // ¼ c sweetener, such as stevia or swerve
- ◆ 2 tsp baking powder
- ◆ 1 tsp salt
- ◆ 2 tsp cinnamon
- ◆ 4 large eggs, yolks and whites separated
- ◆ 220g // ½ c butter
- ◆ 1 tsp vanilla extract

DIRECTIONS

1. Start by turning your waffle iron on high and leaving it to heat up. Sieve your flour, sweetener, baking powder, cinnamon, and salt into a large bowl

2. Place your butter into a microwave proof bowl or mug and heat for 20 second intervals until melted, then pour this and your egg yolks into the flour mix and stir to thoroughly combine. In a separate bowl beat your egg whites with a handheld whisk until they form stiff peaks. Fold the egg whites into your batter, being careful to keep in as much air as possible

3. Grease your heated waffle iron and pour in half of your batter. Cook for 5 minutes, or until crisp and golden, then repeat using your remaining batter. Serve your waffles warm, and topped with sugar free maple syrup, butter, cream cheese, or whatever else your favourite toppings may be

CHAFFLES

SERVES	4
CARBOHYDRATES	2G
PROTEIN	20G
FAT	26G
CALORIES	327

INGREDIENTS

♦ 2 tbsp butter
♦ 4 medium eggs
♦ 225g // 2c grated cheddar cheese
♦ 4 tbsp almond flour
♦ Salt and pepper to taste

DIRECTIONS

1. Start by turning your waffle iron on high and leaving it to heat up. Place your butter into a medium sized, microwave proof bowl, and heat on high for 10-20 seconds until your butter is melted. Add in the rest of your ingredients and stir thoroughly to combine

2. Grease your heated waffle iron and pour in a quarter of your batter. Cook for 4-6 minutes, or until golden and crispy, then repeat this process a further 3 times to use up your remaining batter

3. Serve your chaffles warm, and topped with sugar free maple syrup, butter, cream cheese, or whatever else your favourite toppings may be

Tofu Scramble

SERVES	2
CARBOHYDRATES	3.8G
PROTEIN	20.3G
FAT	13.1G
CALORIES	206

INGREDIENTS

- 220g // 1c tofu, firm
- 1tbsp butter
- 2tbsp nutritional yeast
- ½ tsp turmeric
- ½ tsp ground cumin
- ½ tsp garlic powder
- ¼ tsp onion powder
- 60ml // 1/4 c milk

DIRECTIONS

1. Place your tofu in a medium bowl and mash unevenly with a fork- leave some chunks for texture, but nothing too big. Add your seasonings to the bowl and mix gently, being careful to not break your tofu up and further. Once combined pour in the soya milk, and once again mix gently

2. In a medium pan melt your butter. Once melted spoon the tofu, leaving most of the liquid in the bowl. Fry the tofu until lightly browned, then slowly pour in the remaining liquid whilst stirring. The tofu will absorb the liquid, so keep on the heat until your desired consistency is reached

3. Transfer to a plate and serve, topping with fried tomatoes and avocado, or on top of our keto cauliflower bread

Lemon and Blueberry Muffins

SERVES	12
CARBOHYDRATES	6G
PROTEIN	7G
FAT	23G
CALORIES	244

INGREDIENTS

- 360g // 3c almond flour
- 120ml // ½ c melted butter
- 3 large eggs
- 1tbsp lemon zest
- 1 tsp vanilla extract
- 50g // ¼ c sweetener, such as stevia or swerve
- 1 tsp baking powder
- ¼ tsp salt
- 50g // 1/3 c blueberries
- 2 tbsp lemon juice
- Extra lemon zest to serve

DIRECTIONS

1. Before starting preheat your oven to 180C // 350F and line a 12 hole muffin or cupcake tray

2. Place your flour, melted butter, eggs, lemon zest, vanilla extract, sweetener, baking powder, and salt into a large bowl. Using a wooden spoon or handheld mixer beat everything together until it has formed a thick batter. Gently mix in your blueberries, using a wooden spoon to avoid bursting or crushing them

3. Divide the batter equally between your 12 lined holes before placing into the centre of your preheated oven. Bake for 15-20 minutes, or until firm and with some colour, checking they are done by pricking with a skewer that will come out clean

4. Remove the muffins from the oven and leave to cool slightly before brushing with lemon juice and decorating with more lemon zest

COCONUT AND CASHEW BREAKFAST BARS

SERVES	6
CARBOHYDRATES	7G
PROTEIN	5G
FAT	33G
CALORIES	327

INGREDIENTS

♦ 60g // ½ c cashew nuts
♦ 120g // ½ c cashew butter
♦ 60ml // ¼ c coconut oil
♦ 6 tbsp desiccated coconut
♦ 50g // ¼ sweetener, such as stevia or swerve

DIRECTIONS

1. Start by lining a 9x9 baking tin with parchment paper. Place your cashew nuts into a food processor and pulse on high until they are crushed, but retaining texture. Alternatively crush them by hand by placing the nuts into a Ziploc bag and gently hitting with a rolling pin

2. Pour your cashew butter, coconut oil, and desiccated coconut into a medium mixing bowl and stir to thoroughly combine. Add your crushed nuts and sweetener before stirring again. A thick batter should form

3. Pour the batter into the prepared baking tin and use the back of a spoon to spread the mixture evenly, ensuring that all corners of the tin are filling

4. Chill in the fridge for at least an hour (preferably overnight) before cutting into 6 and serving

Bulletproof Coffee

SERVES	1
CARBOHYDRATES	0G
PROTEIN	1G
FAT	38G
CALORIES	334

INGREDIENTS

- 1 cup of freshly brewed coffee
- 2 tbsp unsalted butter
- 1 tbsp coconut oil
- 1 tsp sweetener (if desired)
- A dash of milk (if desired)

DIRECTIONS

1. Pour all your ingredients into a food processor. Blend on high for 20-30 seconds, until the drink is aerated and frothy. Transfer to a mug and serve immediately, adding sweetener or milk to your liking

Granola

SERVES	10
CARBOHYDRATES	7G
PROTEIN	16G
FAT	29G
CALORIES	357

INGREDIENTS

- 110g // ¾ c almonds, pecans, hazelnuts, or any other nuts
- 35g // 1/3 c desiccated coconut
- 150g // 1c mixed pumpkin, sesame, and sunflower seeds
- 8 tbsp flaxseed
- 2 tsp turmeric
- 1 tsp nutmeg
- 2 tsp cinnamon
- 50g // ¼ c almond flour
- 2 tbsp coconut oil

DIRECTIONS

1. Before starting preheat your oven to 150C // 300F and line a large baking tray with parchment paper

2. Place your nuts into a food processor and pulse on high until they are crushed, but retaining texture. Alternatively crush them by hand by placing the nuts into a Ziploc bag and gently hitting with a rolling pin

3. Transfer the crushed nuts to a large mixing bowl, then add all your remaining ingredients and stir with a wooden spoon to mix thoroughly. Pour the mix onto your prepared baking tray and spread it out evenly before placing into the preheated oven

4. Roast the mix for 20 mins, stir, then return to the oven for a further 15-20 minutes. When the granola is starting to turn golden brown and crispy turn off the oven, but do not remove it. Leave the mix in the cooling oven for another 20-30 minutes to cool

5. Store the granola in an airtight container. Serve with Greek yoghurt or coconut cream, or use it as a topping for other dishes

Mains

VEGETARIAN

CAULIFLOWER RICE

SERVES	6
CARBOHYDRATES	13.4G
PROTEIN	5.2G
FAT	0.8G
CALORIES	67

INGREDIENTS

♦ 700g // 2½ c cauliflower florets
  (around 1 large cauliflower head)

DIRECTIONS

1. Chop your cauliflower into florets, trying to leave as little stalk as possible

2. Transfer the florets into a food processor and pulse until broken down and sandy in texture- you may have to do this in batches dependent upon your food processor size. Be careful not to blend too much or you will instead make cauliflower mash

3. Serve raw, or cook in 1tbsp of oil over a medium heat until softened

ROASTED CABBAGE STEAKS

SERVES	5
CARBOHYDRATES	11G
PROTEIN	12G
FAT	16G
CALORIES	243

INGREDIENTS

- 1 small cabbage head
- 120g // ½ c green basil pesto
- 90g // 1c grated parmesan
- 60g // ½ c feta, crumbled
- 2 tsp mixed herbs
- 1 tsp fresh rosemary
- 1 tsp garlic powder
- 10 small plum tomatoes
- 5 marinated artichoke hearts
- 2 tbsp fresh basil, finely sliced

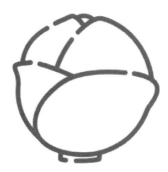

DIRECTIONS

1. Before starting preheat your oven to 200C // 400F and grease a large baking tray. Cut the bottom off your cabbage head (this will make it easier to slice) before taking a large serrated knife and cutting your cabbage into 5 'steaks', roughly 2 cm thick

2. Arrange your cabbage steaks on the baking tray, then divide your pesto between them. Spread the pesto to form a base, then sprinkle over your parmesan, feta, mixed herbs, rosemary, and garlic powder

3. Halve your plum tomatoes and artichoke hearts, then arrange these on top of your covered steaks. Place the baking tray into the preheated oven and bake for 15-20 minutes, or until the cheese has melted and the cabbage is starting to brown at the edges

4. Remove the baking tray from the oven and transfer your steaks to individual plates, before sprinkling over your fresh basil and serving

LOADED CAULIFLOWER CHEESE

SERVES	4
CARBOHYDRATES	7.4G
PROTEIN	11.6G
FAT	24.6G
CALORIES	298

INGREDIENTS

- ♦ 450g // 4c cauliflower florets
- ♦ 120 ml // ½ c sour cream
- ♦ 1 tsp smoked paprika
- ♦ 1 tsp garlic powder
- ♦ 3 tbsp butter
- ♦ 110g // ½ c grated mozzarella
- ♦ 110g // ½ c grated cheddar
- ♦ 1 tsp fresh chilli, sliced
- ♦ Salt and pepper to taste
- ♦ Extra chilli for garnish

DIRECTIONS

1. Before starting preheat your oven to 200C // 400F

2. Bring a large saucepan of salted water to the boil. Boil your cauliflower for 5-10 minutes, or until cooked and softened. Drain the water and leave your cauliflower to cool for a couple of minutes, then transfer to a kitchen towel or cheesecloth and firmly squeeze out any excess liquid

3. Place your cauliflower, sour cream, paprika, garlic powder, and butter in a food processor. Blend until everything is combined, and the cauliflower mix resembles mashed potatoes. Transfer the mix to a baking dish and stir in your sliced chilli and half of your grated cheeses

4. Sprinkle over the remaining half of your grated cheeses and season with salt and pepper, then transfer to your preheated oven. Bake for 5-10 minutes, or until the cheese is melted and bubbling. If you want your cheese to go crispy bake for a further 5 minutes

5. Remove your cauliflower cheese from the oven and sprinkle over a little extra sliced chilli to garnish, then serve immediately

Egg and Blue Cheese Salad

SERVES	6
CARBOHYDRATES	5.1G
PROTEIN	12G
FAT	40.5G
CALORIES	444

INGREDIENTS

- ◆ 8 hard-boiled eggs
- ◆ 60g // ½ c blue cheese
- ◆ 12 cherry tomatoes
- ◆ 1 avocado
- ◆ 3 tbsp full fat mayo
- ◆ 3 tbsp full fat Greek yoghurt
- ◆ 2 tbsp red wine vinegar
- ◆ Salt and pepper to season
- ◆ 2 tbsp fresh chives, chopped

DIRECTIONS

1. First, prepare your ingredients. Do this by cutting your egg into eighths, halving or quartering your tomatoes, crumbling your blue cheese, and cutting your avocado into small chunks, roughly 1cm each. Place all your prepared ingredients into a serving bowl

2. Make the dressing by mixing your mayo, yoghurt, and vinegar in a small bowl. Season with salt and pepper, then pour over the other ingredients in your serving bowl. Lightly toss everything together, then season once again with salt and pepper

3. Sprinkle over your freshly chopped chives, and serve as either a light main or a side dish

Zoodle Alfredo

SERVES	4
CARBOHYDRATES	8G
PROTEIN	26.2G
FAT	55.8G
CALORIES	650

INGREDIENTS

- ◆ 1 shallot, chopped
- ◆ 3 tbsp garlic, minced
- ◆ 60ml // ¼ c white wine
- ◆ 370ml // 1½ c double cream
- ◆ 2 dried bay leaves
- ◆ 60g // ½ c grated parmesan
- ◆ 450g // 3c zoodles
- ◆ Salt and pepper to taste

DIRECTIONS

1. Heat a dash of oil in a large frying pan. Add your shallots and minced garlic, then cook until softened and aromatic- roughly 3 minutes. Pour in your white wine and leave to simmer

2. Once the wine has reduced by roughly half pour in your double cream and bay leaves. Bring to the mixture to a boil and stir continuously until the sauce begins to thicken. Reduce the heat to low and pour in your grated parmesan, then season with salt and pepper. Stir until the parmesan has melted into the sauce

3. Remove the bay leaves from the sauce before adding in the zoodles. Toss the zoodles in the sauce so they are fully coated, the remove the pan from the heat. Serve the pasta warm, topping with additional grated parmesan and a generous sprinkling of cracked black pepper

Portobello Mushroom Tacos

SERVES	6
CARBOHYDRATES	8G
PROTEIN	5G
FAT	17.2G
CALORIES	203

INGREDIENTS

- ♦ 6 large portobello mushrooms, washed and with the stems removed
- ♦ 60g // ¼ c harissa paste
- ♦ 1 tsp ground cumin
- ♦ ½ tsp cayenne pepper
- ♦ 1 tsp onion powder
- ♦ 3 tbsp olive oil
- ♦ 1 large avocado, sliced
- ♦ 1 small red onion, diced
- ♦ 2 tbsp fresh coriander, chopped
- ♦ 6 large lettuce, cabbage, or kale leaves

DIRECTIONS

1. In a small bowl mix together your harissa paste, cumin, cayenne pepper, onion powder, and 1 ½ tbsp of olive oil until fully combined. Cover each mushroom in this harissa marinade and set aside for 10 minutes

2. After 10 minutes heat your remaining oil in a large frying pan. Fry each mushroom for 2 minutes each side, or until slightly softened and browned. Remove the mushrooms from the heat and set aside

3. Prepare your 'tacos' by putting a few slices of avocado along the stem of each leaf. Sprinkle over some of the diced red onion and some of the chopped coriander

4. Slice each mushroom and place it in the prepared leaves. Serve your tacos topped with additional ingredients, for example salsa, cashew cream, or fresh chillies

Pizza Omelette

SERVES	4
CARBOHYDRATES	8G
PROTEIN	48G
FAT	53G
CALORIES	709

INGREDIENTS

- ◆ 8 eggs
- ◆ 8 tbsp cream cheese
- ◆ 3 tsp garlic, minced
- ◆ 600g // 5c grated mozzarella
- ◆ 6 tbsp tomato puree
- ◆ 1 tsp dried basil
- ◆ 2 tsp dried oregano
- ◆ 2 tbsp fresh basil, sliced

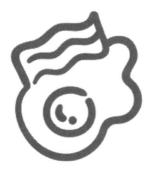

DIRECTIONS

1. Start by preheating your oven to 200C // 400F and lining a large pie dish, or circular baking tin with parchment paper

2. In a large bowl mix together your eggs, cream cheese, minced garlic, and half of your grated mozzarella until thoroughly combined. Press this dough into your prepared dish, being sure to press it evenly, and fully into the corners. Transfer the dish to your preheated oven and cook for 10-15 minutes, or until the base is golden brown and crispy

3. Remove the base from the oven. Spread your tomato puree evenly over the base, then top with the remaining grated mozzarella, dried basil, and dried oregano. Return the pizza to the oven for a further 10-15 minutes, or until the cheese is melted and starting to bubble

4. Remove the pizza from the oven and leave it to cool for a couple of minutes before slicing into quarters. Sprinkle over your fresh basil and serve

Kale, Pomegranate, and Goats Cheese Salad

SERVES	4
CARBOHYDRATES	7G
PROTEIN	11G
FAT	29G
CALORIES	331

INGREDIENTS

- 200g // 1½ c chopped kale
- ¼ pomegranate, seeds removed
- 120g // 1c goats cheese, crumbled
- 60ml // ¼ c olive oil
- 2 tsp Dijon mustard
- 1 tbsp balsamic vinegar
- 2 tbsp fresh orange juice
- Salt and pepper to taste
- 3 tbsp pumpkin seeds

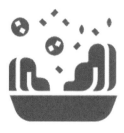

DIRECTIONS

1. Make the salad dressing by pouring your olive oil, Dijon mustard, balsamic vinegar, and orange juice into a small bowl and whisking until combined

2. Wash your kale and remove any obvious stems. Place your kale into a large serving bowl. Pour over your dressing and toss everything together to coat the leaves in dressing

3. Add your pomegranate seeds and goats cheese before seasoning with salt and pepper. Toss everything once again to distribute the ingredients throughout the salad

4. Sprinkle over the pumpkin seeds to garnish. Serve as either a light main or a side dish

BAKED BRIE

SERVES	4
CARBOHYDRATES	1G
PROTEIN	15G
FAT	31G
CALORIES	342

INGREDIENTS

- ♦ 1 medium brie wheel
- ♦ 1 small yellow onion, sliced
- ♦ 2 tbsp balsamic vinegar
- ♦ 2 tbsp garlic, minced
- ♦ 1 tbsp olive oil
- ♦ 2 tbsp fresh rosemary, chopped
- ♦ 3 tbsp walnuts, finely chopped

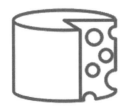

DIRECTIONS

1. Start by preheating your oven to 200C // 400F and lining a small baking tray with parchment paper

2. Heat a small frying pan on a medium heat. Once hot, pour in your sliced onions, balsamic vinegar, and 2 tbsp of water. Cover the pan and sauté the onions for 2-4 minutes, shaking the pan to ensure the onions don't burn. Once softened remove from the heat and set aside

3. Place your garlic, olive oil, and rosemary in a small bowl. Heat in the microwave for 2 seconds, then remove from the microwave and add in your finely chopped walnuts, stirring to ensure the walnuts are coated

4. Place your brie wheel onto the prepared baking tray. Take a sharp knife and make a few small scores all over the cheese. Place your sauteed onions in the centre of the cheese, then pour over your oil and nut mix

5. Transfer the baking tray to the preheated oven and bake the cheese for 10-15 minutes, or until the cheese is warm and aromatic. Remove from the oven and serve immediately, pairing with low carb crackers, roasted vegetables, or nuts for dipping

MEAT

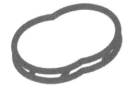

ICEBERG BURGERS

SERVES	4
CARBOHYDRATES	7.9G
PROTEIN	8.7G
FAT	8.6G
CALORIES	311

INGREDIENTS

- 500g // 2c beef mince
- 1 tbsp mixed herbs
- 1 tbsp garlic, minced
- 1 tsp black pepper
- 1 tsp salt
- 1 tsp oil
- 4 Slices of bacon
- 1 white or yellow onion, sliced
- 1 large head of iceberg lettuce
- 1 large tomato
- 4 slices of cheese, preferably cheddar or mozzarella

DIRECTIONS

1. Place your beef mince into a large bowl and add your mixed herbs, garlic, black pepper, and salt. Using your hands or a wooden spoon, mix everything together until thoroughly combined, then divide the mix into 4 and shape each portion into a burger patty. Set aside

2. Heat 1tsp of oil in a large pan and fry your bacon until it is brown and crispy, then transfer to a paper towel lined plate. Using the same pan, turn the heat to medium and cook your burger patties. Cook the patties for about 4 minutes each side, or to your preference, the place a slice of cheese on each cooked burger. Turn off the heat and place a lid on the pan to melt the cheese

3. Whilst the cheese melts take your lettuce head and cut 8 rounds from your lettuce head to form 'buns', and slice your tomato into slices

4. Assemble your burgers by placing a slice of tomato on the bottom 'bun'. Add your burger and a rasher of bacon, then top with another lettuce round 'bun'. Serve your burgers drizzled with ranch, tomato, or burger sauce

HERBY LAMB CHOPS

SERVES	4
CARBOHYDRATES	0.1G
PROTEIN	21G
FAT	31G
CALORIES	362

INGREDIENTS

♦ 120g // ½ c butter
♦ 2 tbsp garlic, minced
♦ 4 tbsp fresh parsley, finely chopped
♦ 4 lamb chops
♦ 1 tbsp olive oil
♦ 1 lemon, cut into 6
♦ Salt and pepper to taste

DIRECTIONS

1. Remove your chops from the fridge and set them aside to reach room temperature, and whilst they acclimatise make your herb butter. Do this by placing your butter, garlic, and parsley in a small bowl, and season with salt and pepper. Use a handheld whisk to beat the butter until all ingredients are fully combined, then set aside to infuse

2. Rub your chops with salt and pepper, and heat your olive oil in a medium frying pan. Fry each chop for 2-3 minutes each side, adjusting times depending upon the thickness of the chops

3. Transfer the chops to plates and squeeze over a little lemon juice. Divide the herb butter between the 4 chops, then serve garnished with a slice of lemon

Grilled Salmon

SERVES	4
CARBOHYDRATES	1G
PROTEIN	79G
FAT	26G
CALORIES	570

INGREDIENTS

- 4 salmon fillets
- 1 lemon
- 2 tbsp garlic, minced
- 1 tbsp fresh rosemary, finely chopped
- 1 tbsp fresh thyme, finely chopped
- 1 shallot, finely chopped
- 1 tbsp Dijon mustard
- Salt and pepper to taste

DIRECTIONS

1. Start by setting your grill to medium and leaving it to heat, then line a medium baking tray with parchment paper and arrange your salmon fillets on top

2. Place your garlic, rosemary, thyme, shallot, and mustard in a small bowl. Halve your lemon and squeeze in the juice from one half. Stir everything together, before seasoning with salt and pepper, and stirring again

3. Brush the mixture over the fillets, then place them under the grill for 6-8 minutes, or until pink and cooked

4. Transfer the salmon to plates. Cut your remaining lemon half into quarters, and serve each fillet with a slice of lemon

FRIED CHICKEN AND BROCCOLI

SERVES	2
CARBOHYDRATES	5G
PROTEIN	29G
FAT	66G
CALORIES	733

INGREDIENTS

- 1 medium broccoli head
- 60g // ½ c butter
- 4 chicken breasts
- ½ tsp smoked paprika
- ½ tsp onion powder
- 1 tsp garlic, minced
- ½ tsp dried thyme
- ½ tsp dried rosemary
- 1 tsp dried basil
- 125ml // ½ c mayonnaise
- 2 tbsp lemon juice

DIRECTIONS

1. Prepare your broccoli by cutting into medium florets and washing. Set the broccoli aside to dry, and in the meantime place your paprika, onion powder, garlic, thyme, rosemary, and basil into a small bowl. Stir to thoroughly combine, then rub this spice mix all over your chicken breasts

2. Heat half of your butter in a large frying pan. Add your chicken breasts and fry for roughly 5 minutes each side, or until aromatic, golden brown, and cooked through

3. Add the rest of your butter and allow it to melt before pouring in your prepared broccoli. Season with salt and pepper, then fry for a further 4-6 minutes, or until the broccoli is softened to your liking

4. Mix your mayonnaise and lemon juice to thin the mayonnaise. Place a chicken breast on each plate and divide up the broccoli evenly, before drizzling with the mayonnaise and serving

Tuna Burgers

SERVES	8
CARBOHYDRATES	8G
PROTEIN	39G
FAT	79G
CALORIES	911

INGREDIENTS

- 700g // 3c canned tuna
- 80g // 1/3 c almond flour
- 2 medium green onions, finely chopped
- 2tbsp chopped dill
- zest of 1 lemon
- ½ tsp salt
- ½ tsp pepper
- 75ml // ¼ c mayonnaise
- 1 large egg
- 1 tbsp lemon juice
- 2 tbsp oil

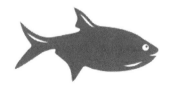

DIRECTIONS

1. Combine tuna, flour, egg, and mayonnaise in a large bowl, then add the onion, dill, lemon juice and zest, and season with salt and pepper. Stir again, making sure everything is thoroughly combined

2. Shape the mixture to form 8 patties, then leave them to rest in the fridge for 10 minutes

3. Heat oil in a large non-stick frying pan, then add your patties- cook for around 4 minutes each side, or until browned and crispy. Once fried place on a plate covered with a paper towel to remove any excess oil

4. Serve with leafy greens, lemon, and capers

Chicken and Greens Soup

SERVES	6
CARBOHYDRATES	12G
PROTEIN	33G
FAT	31G
CALORIES	455

INGREDIENTS

- ◆ 3tbsp butter
- ◆ 1 large yellow onion, finely chopped
- ◆ 2 tbsp fresh ginger, finely chopped
- ◆ 2 tbsp garlic, minced
- ◆ 450g // 3c cauliflower florets
- ◆ 250g // 1½ c cream cheese
- ◆ 1 litre // 4c chicken stock
- ◆ 275g // 2c kale
- ◆ 450g // 3c cooked chicken, shredded
- ◆ Salt and pepper to taste
- ◆ 3 tbsp pumpkin seeds

DIRECTIONS

1. Heat the butter in a large, heavy bottomed pan over a medium heat. Once the butter has melted add in your onion, ginger, garlic, and cauliflower, and sauté for 4-6 minutes, or until all the ingredients are softened

2. Reduce the heat to low and pour in your cream cheese. Stir until the cream cheese is completely melted, then season with salt and pepper. Pour in the chicken stock and kale, and leave on a high heat for 3-5 minutes

3. Transfer the soup to a food processor and blend until smooth and creamy, then return to the pan. Bring the soup to the boil, then reduce to a steady simmer. Leave the soup to simmer for 5-10 minutes before pouring in your shredded chicken

4. Divide the soup between 6 bowls, then top with a sprinkling of pumpkin seeds and serve piping hot

STEAK STIR FRY

SERVES	2
CARBOHYDRATES	10G
PROTEIN	42G
FAT	77G
CALORIES	893

INGREDIENTS

- 2 Ribeye steaks
- ½ tsp salt
- 1 tsp black pepper
- 120g // 1c butter
- 1 tbsp fresh ginger, finely chopped
- 2 tbsp garlic, minced
- 1 medium yellow onion, sliced
- 1 small broccoli head, cut into florets
- 1 tbsp tamari soy sauce
- 2 tbsp peanuts, roughly chopped
- 1 chilli, finely chopped

DIRECTIONS

1. Prepare your meat by slicing the steak into strips, roughly 2cm thick. Heat half of your butter in a wok on a medium heat, then add in your steak strips fry until browned. Once cooked remove the steak from the wok and set aside

2. Add another 2tbsp of butter to the wok and allow it to melt before adding in your ginger, garlic, sliced onion, and broccoli florets. Fry for 3-5 minutes, or until the onion and broccoli are softened. Return your steak strips to the pan and add in the soy sauce

3. Reheat the steak strips and season with salt and pepper, tossing the stir fry to ensure everything is coated with sauce

4. Once everything is heated and cooked divide the mixture evenly between two serving dishes. Sprinkle over the chopped peanuts and chilli to serve

Chicken Chilli

SERVES	4
CARBOHYDRATES	10.5G
PROTEIN	27G
FAT	16.5G
CALORIES	302

INGREDIENTS

- 4 chicken breasts
- 1 tbsp butter
- 1 large white onion, sliced
- 500ml // 2c chicken stock
- 250ml // 1c tinned tomatoes
- 2 tbsp tomato puree
- 1 tbsp chilli powder
- 1 tsp smoked paprika
- 2 tsp cumin
- 1 tsp turmeric
- 2 tsp garlic powder
- 110g // 2/3 c cream cheese
- 2 tbsp fresh coriander, finely chopped

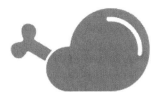

DIRECTIONS

1. In a large, heavy bottomed pan melt your butter, then add in your onion and sauté until it is softened. Pour in your chicken stock, tinned tomatoes, tomato puree, chilli powder, paprika, cumin, turmeric, and garlic powder, and leave to simmer on a low heat

2. Whilst your sauce simmers prepare your chicken; heat a large frying pan, arranging your chicken breasts inside. Pour boiling water into the pan, covering the chicken, but only just. Leave this to boil for 10 minutes, or until the chicken is cooked through. Remove the breasts from the pan

3. Using two forks, shred your chicken breasts and add the shredded meat to your tomato sauce. Bring the sauce to a boil and add in your cream cheese, stirring until it is fully melted and incorporated. Leave to simmer for another couple of minutes

4. Divide the chicken chilli between 4 bowls. Finish with a sprinkling of fresh coriander, or grated cheese if desired, and serve piping hot

PORK CHOPS WITH BLUE CHEESE SAUCE

SERVES	4
CARBOHYDRATES	4G
PROTEIN	54G
FAT	60G
CALORIES	779

INGREDIENTS

- 150g // 1c blue cheese, crumbled
- 175ml // ¾ c double cream
- 2 tbsp walnuts, crushed
- 4 pork chops
- 2 tbsp olive oil
- Freshly cracked black pepper

DIRECTIONS

1. Place your blue cheese into a small saucepan and place it over a low heat, stirring regularly to avoid any burning whilst it melts. Once melted pour in the double cream and increase the heat. Simmer for 5 minutes, then remove from the heat and stir in your crushed walnuts

2. Heat your olive oil in a large frying pan, then add in the pork chops and fry for 2-3 minutes on each side. Once cooked through remove the chops from the heat. Pour any liquid into the sauce, then cover the pan with foil and set aside

3. Return the sauce to the heat for a couple of minutes, stirring to mix in any juices from the chops. Once the sauce is adequately hot transfer your chops to plates and divide the sauce evenly between each portion. Serve accompanied by fresh vegetables and with a generous topping of freshly cracked black pepper

Ham Croquettes

SERVES	4
CARBOHYDRATES	2G
PROTEIN	34G
FAT	131G
CALORIES	1342

INGREDIENTS

- ◆ 450g // 3c cured ham, diced
- ◆ 1 tsp garlic powder
- ◆ 1 tsp onion powder
- ◆ 4 tbsp fresh oregano, finely sliced
- ◆ 4 tbsp fresh basil, finely sliced
- ◆ 4 tbsp fresh rosemary, finely sliced
- ◆ 4 egg whites
- ◆ 100g // 1c almond flour
- ◆ 475 ml // 2c coconut oil

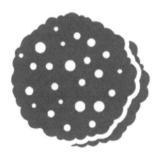

DIRECTIONS

1. Place your ham, garlic powder, onion powder, oregano, basil, rosemary, and 1 egg white into a food processor. Blend on high for 30-60 seconds, or until all ingredients are fully blended, and have formed a thick, doughy texture

2. Heat your coconut oil in a medium, heavy bottomed pan. Whilst the oil heats and melts divide your ham mixture into 8 or 12 (depending on how large you wan your croquettes) and shape each portion into a ball

3. Having your egg whites and almond flour ready in separate bowls, dip each croquette into the egg whites and then into the almond flour. Repeat this so each croquette will be dipped twice in both, then drop the croquettes into the heated coconut oil

4. Fry each croquette for 6 minutes, being sure to move them around the pan so all sides are equally golden and crispy. Transfer them to a paper towel lined plate to cool for a couple of minutes before serving

Spicy Shrimp Skewers

SERVES	4
CARBOHYDRATES	2G
PROTEIN	16G
FAT	11G
CALORIES	176

INGREDIENTS

- ♦ 450g // 3½ c large shrimps
- ♦ 3 tbsp butter, melted
- ♦ 2 tbsp harissa paste
- ♦ 1 tsp cayenne pepper
- ♦ 1 tsp ground cumin
- ♦ 1 tbsp fresh lime juice
- ♦ 2 tbsp garlic, minced
- ♦ Salt and pepper to taste
- ♦ 1 lime, quartered
- ♦ 1 tbsp fresh coriander, finely chopped

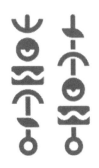

DIRECTIONS

1. Before starting be sure to peel and devein your shrimp. After doing so, season them with salt and pepper and set aside

2. In a medium bowl mix together your melted butter, harissa paste, cayenne pepper, cumin, lime juice, and garlic. Season with salt and pepper, then pour in your shrimp. Toss the shrimp to ensure all are evenly covered, and preferably leave to marinade for at least 30 minutes

3. After the shrimp have marinated divide them equally between 4 skewers, leaving a small gap between each shrimp on the skewer

4. Place a large frying pan over a high heat. Once the pan is hot add the skewers, cooking for 2-3 minutes on each side, or until fully cooked through

5. Transfer the skewers to plates, and serve finished with a lime wedge and a sprinkling of coriander

EXCLUSIVE BONUS

40 Weight Loss Recipes

&

14 Days Meal Plan

Scan the QR-Code and receive
the FREE download:

2 WEEK KETO KICKSTARTER MEAL PLAN

Featuring recipes from the book, and a new and exciting breakfast, lunch, or dinner daily, this meal plan is a great way to start your keto journey.

The recipes that follow are proof that dieting doesn't need to be boring, and it certainly isn't just salad!

Enjoy the coming two weeks by kickstart your new keto lifestyle today

DAY 1

BREAKFAST: GRANOLA (SEE PAGE 39)

LUNCH: AVOCADO, SPINACH AND FETA CHEESE FRITTATA

SERVES	6
CARBOHYDRATES	3G
PROTEIN	12G
FAT	18G
CALORIES	231

INGREDIENTS

- 1 bag // 4 c spinach
- ½ brown onion
- 8 eggs
- 1 tbsp milk
- 1 large avocado (diced)
- 120g // ¾ c feta cheese (crumbled)
- oil

DIRECTIONS

1. Before starting preheat your oven to 200C // 400F and oil a large baking dish

2. Sautee onion and spinach in an oiled pan until the onion is soft and the spinach is wilted, then transfer them into the oiled dish

3. In another bowl whisk eggs until foamy, adding the salt and pepper for taste. Pour the eggs over the vegetables into the dish

4. Place into the oven and cook for 5 minutes, or until the edges have started to set. At this stage add the diced avocado, evenly sprinkling it over the dish

5. Cook for a further 5 minutes before crumbling the feta evenly over the dish. Having added both your feta and avocado cook for a further 5 minutes, or until the mixture is golden brown and cooked through

6. Allow to cool for a couple of minutes before serving

DINNER: PIZZA OMELETTE (SEE PAGE 54)

DAY 2

Breakfast: Oatmeal

SERVES	1
CARBOHYDRATES	8G
PROTEIN	10G
FAT	61G
CALORIES	615

INGREDIENTS

♦ 110ml // ½ c coconut or almond milk (unsweetened)

♦ 2 tsp flaxseed

♦ 2 tsp chia seeds

♦ 1tsp sunflower seeds

♦ pinch of salt

♦ ½ tsp vanilla extract

DIRECTIONS

1. Heat the milk, sunflower seeds, flaxseeds and chia in a small saucepan. Bring the mixture to a boil before turning the heat to medium, and stirring in salt and vanilla extract to taste

2. Keep the mixture on the heat, stirring occasionally, until your desired consistency is reached

3. Transfer to a bowl and serve with a sprinkling of cinnamon, more seeds, or coconut cream

LUNCH: TUNA BURGERS (SEE PAGE 67)

DINNER: ZOODLE ALFREDO (SEE PAGE 50)

DAY 3

Breakfast: Chaffles (See page 32)
Lunch: Grilled Salmon (See page 64)
Dinner : Chicken nuggets

SERVES	4
NET CARBS	6G
FIBER	2G
FAT	74G
PROTEIN	41G
CALORIES	869

INGREDIENTS

- 500g // 4c boneless chicken breast or thighs, cut into bite sized pieces
- 75g // ½ c shredded parmesan cheese
- ½ tsp onion powder
- 1 egg (small)
- Salt and pepper to taste
- 2 tsp oil (we recommend coconut)

BEAN FRIES

- 150g // 1c green beans trimmed
- 2tsp coconut oil

BBQ DIPPING SAUCE

- 125ml // 2/3 c mayonnaise

- ♦ 2 tsp tomato puree
- ♦ ½ tsp smoked paprika
- ♦ ½ tsp garlic powder
- ♦ Salt and pepper to taste

DIRECTIONS

1. Before starting, preheat your oven to 180C//350F and oil a medium baking tray

2. To create the nugget crumb, thoroughly combine the parmesan and onion powder in a medium mixing bowl

3. In a separate bowl whisk the egg until frothy, adding salt and pepper to season

4. Mix your chicken pieces into the egg and make sure that they are evenly coated with egg mixture

5. One at a time remove your chicken pieces from the egg mixture and coat in the nugget crumb, before shaking off any excess and placing evenly spaced on the baking tray. Repeat until all the chicken is used up

6. Bake the chicken in the oven for 15-20 minutes, or until crispy and cooked through. Turn halfway through baking

7. Whilst the chicken is baking make the bean fries by heating the oil in a medium pan over a high heat. Once the oil is melted add the beans and fry for a few minutes so they are crispy- if fried for too long they will soften and wilt

8. Make the dipping sauce by combining all the ingredients in a small bowl, adjusting spice measurements to taste

9. Once the chicken is cooked transfer to plates and serve with the bean fries and BBQ dipping sauce

DAY 4

Breakfast: Eggs Benedict (See page 22)
Lunch: Chicken Chilli (See page 73)
Dinner: Roasted Tomato Tart

SERVES	6
CARBOHYDRATES	6.7G
PROTEIN	22.6G
FAT	29.3G
CALORIES	381

INGREDIENTS

DOUGH

- 100g // 1c almond flour
- 170g //1½ c shredded mozzarella
- 1tbsp (heaped) cream cheese
- 1 egg (large)
- 1tsp onion powder
- ½ tsp garlic powder

FILLING

- 250g // 1½ c cherry tomatoes
- 1 red onion
- 2tbsp fresh basil (chopped)
- 2 eggs (large)
- 2 tbsp ricotta cheese

- 60g // ½ c shredded mozzarella
- 1tbsp olive oil

DIRECTIONS

1. Before starting preheat your oven to 200C//400F and line a baking tray with parchment paper

2. To make the dough heat the shredded mozzarella in the microwave. Do this by placing it in a microwave proof bowl, and heating then stirring at 20 second intervals until fully melted

3. Add the remaining ingredients and mix until it resembles a soft dough

4. Roll into a circle between two sheets of parchment paper- make sure the dough is evenly about 1/2cm thick. Leave the dough to rest

5. Whilst the dough rests start to make the filling- do this by whisking together the eggs and ricotta cheese until smooth, then add the shredded mozzarella, basil, and season with salt and pepper before beating to combine once again

6. Spoon the creamy mixture onto your dough base, being sure to leave a border of 2-3cm. Create a heightened crust by rolling this border inwards

7. Slice the red onion and sprinkle on top of the galette, then oil and add the tomatoes

8. Bake for 15-20 minutes, or until the crust is golden and crisp, and the filling is cooked through, but with a slight wobble in the middle

9. Garnish with fresh basil leaves before serving

DAY 5

Breakfast: Green Smoothie

SERVES	1
CARBOHYDRATES	6G
PROTEIN	2G
FAT	16G
CALORIES	164

INGREDIENTS

- ◆ 75ml // 1/3 c coconut milk
- ◆ 150ml // 2/3 c water
- ◆ 2 tbsp lime juice
- ◆ 170g // ¾ c spinach (preferably frozen)
- ◆ 1tbsp freshly grated ginger
- ◆ 1 tsp desiccated coconut to serve

DIRECTIONS

1. Place coconut milk, water, and spinach into blender and liquidise
2. Add lime juice and ginger to taste
3. Serve cold with a lime wedge and a sprinkle of desiccated coconut

Lunch: Baked Brie (See page 58)

Dinner: Iceberg Burgers (See page 61)

DAY 6

BREAKFAST: CAULIFLOWER TOAST (SEE PAGE 26)

LUNCH: BROCCOLI AND PARMESAN FRITTERS

SERVES	4
CARBOHYDRATES	5.3G
PROTEIN	10.7G
FAT	11.4G
CALORIES	95

INGREDIENTS

- 350g // 1 medium broccoli head
- 4 large eggs
- 35g // 1/3 c almond flour
- 50g // ½ c grated parmesan
- 1 tsp onion powder
- 1 tbsp garlic, minced
- 1 tsp chilli flakes
- Salt and pepper to taste
- 1 tbsp butter
- Chilli flakes to serve

DIRECTIONS

1. Chop the broccoli into florets before placing them into a food processor. Pulse until the broccoli is finely chopped to a sand like consistency

2. Pour the blended broccoli onto a dishtowel or kitchen paper and leave for 10 minutes to remove any excess moisture

3. After the 10 minutes add all your ingredients in a large mixing bowl and stir thoroughly to ensure everything is combined. Leave to stand for a further 10 minutes before stirring once again. Divide the mixture into 4 and shape each ¼ into a fritter

4. Heat your oil in a large non-stick pan. Fry the fritters for about 4 minutes per side, making sure the bottom is cooked and crisp before flipping. Once cooked through transfer to a paper towel lined plate. Once all the fritters are cooked serve them warm and with a sprinkling of chilli flakes

DINNER: HERBY LAMB CHOPS (SEE PAGE 63)

DAY 7

BREAKFAST: COCONUT AND CASHEW BREAKFAST BARS (SEE PAGE 37)
LUNCH: PORTOBELLO MUSHROOM TACOS (SEE PAGE 52)
DINNER: TURKEY AND BELL PEPPER SAUTÉ

SERVES	4
CARBOHYDRATES	11G
PROTEIN	30G
FAT	8G
CALORIES	230

INGREDIENTS

- 450g // 3c turkey tenderloin, cut into 1cm slices
- 1 small onion, sliced
- 1 red bell pepper, sliced
- 1 yellow bell pepper, sliced
- 2 tbsp olive oil
- 1 tsp mixed herbs
- 1 tbsp red wine vinegar
- 125 ml // ½ c tinned tomatoes
- Salt and pepper to taste

DIRECTIONS

1. Heat your oil in a large pan and add in your sliced turkey. Cook for 2-5 minutes, browning both sides and cooking through

2. Add in your onion and peppers, then season with salt and pepper. Cover the pan with a lid and sauté on low for 5-7 minutes, or until the vegetables are softened and starting to brown- be sure to remove the lid and stir every couple of minutes

3. Increase the heat to medium and add in your mixed herbs, vinegar, and tinned tomatoes. Stir everything together and leave to simmer for 5 minutes, or until the sauce has reduced by ¼ - ½

4. Ensure the turkey is hot before serving

DAY 8

BREAKFAST: BULLETPROOF COFFEE (SEE PAGE 38)

LUNCH: CASHEW CHICKEN

SERVES	3
CARBOHYDRATES	8G
PROTEIN	22.6G
FAT	24G
CALORIES	334

INGREDIENTS

- 3 chicken thighs, boneless and deskinned
- 2tbsp coconut oil
- 1 small white onion
- 1 small red pepper
- ½ tsp fresh ginger, finely chopped
- 2 tbsp garlic, minced
- 1 tsp cayenne pepper
- 1tbsp rice wine vinegar
- 1 tbsp soya sauce
- 40g // ¼ c cashew nuts
- Salt and pepper to taste
- 1tbsp sesame seeds
- Sliced green onion

DIRECTIONS

1. Prepare your ingredients by cutting your chicken thighs into 1cm chunks and slicing your onion and pepper. Heat 1tbsp of coconut oil in a large frying pan and add your chopped chicken thighs, cooking for 4-5 minutes, or until slightly brown and cooked through

2. Increase the heat to high and add your remaining coconut oil to the pan, then pour in your onion, pepper, ginger, garlic, and cayenne pepper, and season with salt and pepper. Cook for another 2-3 minutes

3. Add in your vinegar, soya sauce, and cashews, and toss everything together to ensure it is all coated with some sauce, then leave to cook down for 2-4 minutes

4. Transfer to bowls and top with a sprinkling of sesame seed and green onion to serve

DINNER: LOADED CAULIFLOWER CHEESE (SEE PAGE 46)

DAY 9

BREAKFAST: CLOUD EGGS

SERVES	4
CARBOHYDRATES	3.9G
PROTEIN	31G
FAT	20.8G
CALORIES	325

INGREDIENTS

- 120g // 1c grated parmesan
- 250g // 1½ c cured ham, chopped
- 8 large eggs whites
- 4 egg yolks
- Salt and pepper to taste
- Fresh basil to serve

DIRECTIONS

1. Start by preheating your oven to 200C//450F and line a large baking tray with parchment paper, oil lightly oil it

2. Have your egg whites in a large glass bowl, making sure the bowl is thoroughly cleaned beforehand, otherwise the whites will not whisk. Use a handheld whisk and beat the eggs on a high speed for 2-3 minutes, or until they double in size and form stiff white peaks

3. Add your parmesan and ham to your egg whites then season with salt and pepper. Gently fold everything together, being sure to keep as much air in the whites as is possible

4. Divide the mixture into 4 and spoon each portion onto the baking tray, leaving as much space as possible between them. Wet a serving spoon and press the back into each portion to create a small crater, then transfer to the preheated oven for 2-3 minutes

5. Remove the baking try from the oven and place an egg yolk into each crater, then season again with salt and pepper. Return to the oven for a further 3-4 minutes, or until the whites are cooked through and slightly browned and the yolks have set slightly

6. Transfer the eggs to plates and serve garnished with fresh basil

Lunch: Chicken and Greens Soup (See page 69)

Dinner: Roasted Cabbage Steaks (See page 44)

DAY 10

<u>BREAKFAST: HUEVOS RANCHEROS (SEE PAGE 24)</u>

LUNCH: HAM CROQUETTES (SEE PAGE 76)

DINNER : FALAFEL WRAPS

SERVES	4
CARBOHYDRATES	16G
PROTEIN	32G
FAT	103G
CALORIES	1124

INGREDIENTS

- 75g // ½ c sliced almonds
- 75g // ½ c pumpkin seeds
- 225g // 3c mushrooms sliced
- 125ml // ½ c oil (olive or coconut)
- 175ml // ¾ c pea protein powder
- 4 tbsp chia seeds
- 1 tbsp diced garlic
- 1 tbsp coriander finely chopped
- 1 tsp ground cumin
- 1 tsp turmeric
- 1 tbsp onion powder
- 60ml // ¼ c water
- 4 large lettuce, cabbage, or kale leaves
- Salt and pepper to taste

DIRECTIONS

1. Before starting preheat oven to 170C//350F and grease a baking sheet

2. Toast almonds and pumpkin seeds in an unoiled frying pan for 2 minutes, then transfer to a food processor and pulse until they are finely chopped, but still have texture

3. Sautee mushrooms and garlic in 1tbsp of the oil until soft, then transfer them and the remaining ingredients to the food processor. Blend once again, before pouring everything into a large bowl, and mixing by hand to ensure everything is fully combined

4. Divide the mixture into 4 before shaping each portion into 3 balls or sausages. Bake in the preheated oven for 15-20 minutes, or until golden and crispy

5. Remove them from the oven and serve each portion inside a leaf to create a falafel wrap

DAY 11

Breakfast: Cinnamon Rolls

SERVES	4
CARBOHYDRATES	4G
PROTEIN	16G
FAT	25G
CALORIES	307

INGREDIENTS

DOUGH

- 1 tbsp orange juice
- 340g // 1½ c grated mozzarella
- 2 tbsp cream cheese
- 1 medium egg
- 75g // ¾ c almond flour
- 1 tbsp sweetener, such as stevia or swerve

FILLING

- 1 tsp cinnamon
- 1 tsp nutmeg
- 1 tsp ginger
- 1 tbsp sweetener, such as stevia or swerve
- 2 tbsp warm water

ICING

- 1 tbsp cream cheese

- ♦ 1 tbsp Greek Yoghurt
- ♦ 1 tbsp sweetener, such as stevia or swerve

DIRECTIONS

1. Start by preheating your oven to 180C // 350 F. To make the dough place your orange juice, grated mozzarella, and cream cheese into a large, microwave proof bowl, and heat on high for 20 second intervals until melted- this should take around 2 minutes

2. Remove the mixture from the microwave and add in your egg, almond flour, and sweetener, stirring thoroughly to combine. Roll the dough out into a rectangle shape, placing it between two sheets of parchment paper to avoid sticking

3. Transfer the dough to a large baking tray and place in the preheated oven for 5 minutes, before removing and setting aside to cool

4. Whilst your dough cools mix together all your 'filling' ingredients in a small bowl. Spread this over your dough, being sure that the all the dough is covered

5. Starting from one of the long sides roll your dough up to create one long log. Cut this into 4 thick rolls, then arrange on the baking tray and return to the oven. Bake for a further 5-7 minutes, or until firmed and golden

6. Remove the rolls from the oven and leave to cool slightly. Whilst they cool make your icing, mixing together all 'icing' ingredients to form a thick paste. Spread this over the rolls and serve immediately whilst still warm

LUNCH: KALE, POMEGRANATE, AND GOATS CHEESE SALAD (SEE PAGE 56)
DINNER: STEAK STIR FRY (SEE PAGE 71)

DAY 12

BREAKFAST: TOFU SCRAMBLE (SEE PAGE 33)
LUNCH: ASIAN PORK BOWL

SERVES	4
CARBOHYDRATES	11G
PROTEIN	22G
FAT	32G
CALORIES	420

INGREDIENTS

- 1 tbsp butter
- 2 tbsp garlic, minced
- 1 tbsp fresh ginger, finely chopped
- 1 small white onion, sliced
- 450g // 2c ground pork
- 1 medium carrot, grated
- ¼ small cabbage head, sliced
- 1 tbsp rice wine vinegar
- 1 tbsp siracha or chilli sauce
- 60 ml // ¼ c soya sauce
- 2 tbsp peanuts, crushed

DIRECTIONS

1. Heat your butter in a large wok over a medium heat. Add your garlic and ginger, and sauté for 2 minutes, or until browning and aromatic. Add in your onion and sauté for a further 2-3 minutes, or until tender and translucent
2. Add your ground pork to the wok, breaking it up to incorporate the other ingredients. Fry until all the pork is browned, then add in your carrot and cabbage, stirring everything to combine
3. Pour in your vinegar, siracha, and soya sauce, and mix everything together. Cook for a further 5-7 minutes, or until the cabbage is wilted and tender
4. Divide between 4 bowls and serve topped with crushed peanuts

DINNER: PORK CHOPS WITH BLUE CHEESE SAUCE (SEE PAGE 75)

DAY 13

BREAKFAST: BREAKFAST FAT BOMBS

SERVES	8
CARBOHYDRATES	8.6G
PROTEIN	2.7G
FAT	18.9G
CALORIES	204

INGREDIENTS

- 75g // ½ c raspberries
- 225g // 1c cream cheese, left at room temperature to soften
- 60ml // ¼ c coconut oil
- Pinch of salt
- 80g // ½ c Keto friendly chocolate chips

DIRECTIONS

1. Begin by placing your raspberries in a mixing bowl and crushing them with the back of a fork. Add in your cream cheese, half your coconut oil, and salt, and combine everything using a handheld whisk. Place the mixture in the freezer for 5 minutes

2. Whilst the mixture firms line a baking tray with parchment paper. Remove the mixture from the freezer and roll it into 16 equal sized balls. Return to the freezer for 5 minutes

3. As the balls harden melt you r keto friendly chocolate chips. Place them in a microwave proof bowl and add in your remaining coconut oil. Heat on high at 15 second intervals, being sure to stir in between each heating period. Once melted, set aside to cool slightly

4. Remove your balls and combine the with the melted chocolate- dip, drizzle, or pipe the chocolate onto every ball. Place in the fridge for 5-10 minutes, then serve

LUNCH: EGG AND BLUE CHEESE SALAD (SEE PAGE 48)
DINNER: FRIED CHICKEN AND BROCCOLI (SEE PAGE 65)

DAY 14

Breakfast: Lemon and Blueberry Muffins (See page 35)
Lunch: Spicy Shrimp Skewers (See page 78)
Dinner: Spinach and Artichoke Stuffed Chicken

SERVES	4
CARBOHYDRATES	2G
PROTEIN	28G
FAT	17G
CALORIES	288

INGREDIENTS

- 4 large chicken breasts
- 80g // ½ c cream cheese
- 60 ml // ¼ c Greek yoghurt
- 100g // 1/3 c grated mozzarella
- 4 marinated artichoke hearts, washed and roughly chopped
- 2 handfuls fresh spinach, shredded
- 1 tbsp mixed herbs
- 2 tbsp butter
- Salt and pepper to taste

DIRECTIONS

1. Score each chicken breast down the middle using a sharp knife. Carefully cut deeper on either side of the score to create a pocket for the filling, then take a rolling pin to tenderise the meat

2. Combine your cream cheese, mozzarella, chopped artichoke hearts, shredded spinach, and mixed herbs in a large bowl. Season with salt and pepper, then mix thoroughly to ensure everything is combined

3. Divide the filling between 4 and stuff each chicken breast with a portion of the cream cheese mixture. If necessary, take a couple of toothpicks and skewer the hole closed to avoid leakage

4. Heat your butter in a large frying pan. Once melted add your stuffed chicken breasts to the pan, cooking each side for 5-7 minutes to ensure the chicken is golden brown, crispy, and cooked through

5. Transfer the stuffed breasts to plates and serve

EXCLUSIVE BONUS

40 Weight Loss Recipes

&

14 Days Meal Plan

Scan the QR-Code and receive
the FREE download:

DISCLAIMER

This book contains opinions and ideas of the author and is meant to teach the reader informative and helpful knowledge while due care should be taken by the user in the application of the information provided. The instructions and strategies are possibly not right for every reader and there is no guarantee that they work for everyone. Using this book and implementing the information/recipes therein contained is explicitly your own responsibility and risk. This work with all its contents, does not guarantee correctness, completion, quality or correctness of the provided information. Misinformation or misprints cannot be completely eliminated.

Printed in Great Britain
by Amazon

87797225R00064